Strength Training

Essential Lifts and Their Benefits

By: Bring On Fitness

information contained within this document, including, but not limited to, errors, omissions, or inaccuracies.

About Bring On Fitness

Our passion for fitness gave life to **Bring On Fitness**. We started with the goal of helping as many people as we can. To educate, motivate and to help change peoples lives for the better. Bring On Fitness is not only for the fitness enthusiasts, but also for the beginner. We strongly believe nothing is more important than learning the basics and creating a strong foundation in both nutrition - through meal planning, and in exercise - by following a specific plan. This is just as important for the beginner, as it is for the experienced athlete.

We set high standards for ourselves, the information we share, and the products we carry. Our goal is to provide you with exceptional products that suit your needs and the knowledge and motivation to help you work towards and achieve your health and fitness goals.

Keep up to date by liking us on Facebook and Instagram @bringonfitness

And for a complete list of reads and a FREE GIFT check us out at: www.bringonfitness.com

"Our Mission is to have a positive impact in changing peoples lives. We will deliver the best possible fitness and nutrition solutions that will empower people to achieve their health and fitness goals."

Table of Contents

Introduction

It's surprising to hear about the many different opinions people have about losing fat and building muscle – opinions that sound as if they are gospel truth. However, of the many different opinions and science-backed methods for getting in shape and staying there, the most effective way combines three crucial components: nutrition, rest, and exercise. Of those three components, we'll tackle exercise in this book, and for optimum fat burning and muscle building, nothing beats strength training.

In this book, you'll learn what strength training is, how you can benefit much from it and the four essential strength training exercises or lifts and how to do them properly. The focus of this book is on what strength training is and its key benefits, and with the information you'll get here, I believe you can be encouraged – armed with information on the benefits – to start a strength training regimen and begin to get leaner.

So if you're ready, turn the page, and let's begin!

10

Chapter 1 - The "What" and "Why" of Strength Training

Strength training – a.k.a. resistance or weight training – is a type of physical exercise with the goal of to achieving better muscular fitness through muscle-specific exercises that move against an external resistance or weight. These include using free weights (e.g., barbells, dumbbells, kettlebells, etc.), machines (e.g., lat pull down and Smith press machines), or body weight (calisthenics). The main principle that governs strength training programs is the application of a particular amount of load on one's muscles with the intention of overloading them, which will make them adapt to the load over time and cause them to become stronger and bigger.

There are two kinds of strength or resistance training: isometric and isotonic. Isometric resistance training requires muscles to contract against an immovable object. In essence, performing isometric resistance exercises mean contracting your muscles and holding them for an extended period of time in that said position. Isotonic exercises involve contracting your muscles against a moving object and throughout a range of motion, i.e., full or partial.

One of the biggest misconceptions about strength training programs is that they're limited to a select group of people, particularly bodybuilders and power lifters. The truth is that strength training is for everybody. The reason for this is that strength training offers many health benefits for any person of any age and any gender. The primary health benefit of strength training for anyone who commits to it for the rest of his or her life is the ability to minimize the muscle-wasting effects of sarcopenia or the natural tendency of muscles to lose mass over time as a person gets older. It doesn't hurt that a good strength training program can make a person's muscles toned and defined.

Other benefits of a good strength training program include:

1. A Stronger and Fitter Body: This is a no-brainer because the name already suggests it. However, the real reason why this is a benefit is because when you're stronger physically, you can do many things much easier. If you don't continue strength training, you may not be able to do many things on your own by the time you get to your sunset years because with aging comes muscle and strength loss.

2. Muscle Mass and Bone Health Protection: Do you know that people start losing muscle mass by age 30 at an average annual rate of about 3% to 5%? Based on an October 2017 published study in the Journal of Bone and Mineral Research, performing resistance and impact exercises at high intensity for as little as 30 minutes twice a week can help improve bone strength, density, and structure in post-menopausal women who suffer from low bone mass without any side effects. It was also noted that performing high intensity resistance exercises can help improve functional performance for the same demographic.

3. Lose Excess Fat and Keep Them Off: While aerobic exercises are proven to be helpful in upping the ante when it comes to daily calories burned for fat loss, it's not as efficient as anaerobic or strength training exercises. Why? For one, strength training exercises – particularly the essential lifts we'll talk about in this book – can burn more calories within a specific period

of time. This means you can work out for as little as 30 minutes and burn as much calories – and body fat – as performing aerobic exercises for more than 1 hour.

Strength training exercises are also able to keep your resting metabolism higher for a much longer period of time after working out compared to aerobic exercises. This means you can burn more calories and body fat even while at rest! How cool is that, huh?

4. Better Body Movements: Performing strength training exercises regularly can help you improve your posture, muscle coordination, and balance. In a study, it was shown that for older people who were at higher risk of falling due to poor physical function, performing strength training exercises can help bring the said risk down by as much as 40%! This is because balance is highly dependent on how strong the muscles that help you stay on your feet are, so the stronger those muscles are, the better you're able to balance your body.

5. Better Management of Chronic Diseases: Performing strength training exercises have been shown in studies to be helpful in managing conditions related to chronic diseases. For example, strength training can help reduce arthritic pain in the same way medicines can. Moreover, strength training, combined with other lifestyle factors, such as diet, can help improve the management of blood sugar in type-2 diabetics.

6. Better Mood and More Energy: Strength training exercises can help you increase your endorphin levels. Endorphins are also called the "happy hormones" and can help make you feel more energetic. Regular strength training exercises have also been shown to help people sleep better, and better sleep provides more energy the next day.

With all of these benefits, why should you put off a good strength training program? The best time to embark on one is now!

14

Chapter 2 - Components of a Good Strength Training Program

One of the misconceptions about strength or weight training programs is that they are mainly for bodybuilders and power lifters. Another is that a strength training program called by any other name is just as good. The truth is that not all of them are created equal. Some are good, but some are crap. The following are some of the key characteristics of a good strength training program.

The Right Exercises

The key word here is "right," i.e., what you need rather than what you want. Many who embark on a strength training program make the mistake of ditching very effective exercises for relatively flimsy reasons, such as they make them look awkward, they're hard, or they just don't like them. If you look at their physiques, chances are that they're a bit pudgy despite being in the gym practically the whole day.

So what are the right exercises? This will mainly depend on your goal, but four of the most important ones that any good strength training program must have are what we'll cover in latter chapters: squats, deadlifts, overhead presses, and bench presses.

Varying Number of Repetitions

Repetitions refer to the number of times you'll need to execute a particular exercise's movements with every set. If you check out many fitness magazines, don't be surprised to find that the standard repetitions for every set of strength training exercises is between 8 and 12. The lower end of the repetition (also called "rep" or "reps" for short) focuses more on developing power and strength, while the higher end focuses more on developing strength and muscular endurance.

Muscles respond best to varying stimuli, which can be achieved by increasing the weights lifted, the speed at which repetitions are done, and the number of repetitions performed. The key here is to achieve muscular failure by the end of your target number of reps. This means if you choose to focus more on power by choosing to perform eight repetitions per set, you mustn't be able to do a ninth rep on your own. If you choose to do ten repetitions, then you shouldn't be able to do an eleventh one anymore. By changing your target number of repetitions, you'll automatically adjust your working weight and vice versa. So by changing your number of repetitions every now and then, you won't give your muscles the chance to completely adapt to the load you're giving them, and they will continue becoming stronger and denser.

Overload Continuously

As mentioned earlier, muscles have the uncanny ability to adapt to the stresses they're regularly subjected to. That's why you need to change things up regularly. One way of doing so is changing the number of reps. Another important principle to ensure that your muscles don't completely adapt and to continue building strength and mass is the progressive overloading principle. This means that if you want your muscles to continue becoming bigger and stronger, you'll need to subject them to increasing resistance over time. If you don't, your strength and mass gains will eventually plateau.

Proper Form over Weight

I've been in the gym long enough to see many people lift relatively heavy weight and have nothing much to show for doing so. Why? It's because they sacrifice proper form at the altar of their egos by lifting more weight than they can properly work with. In some cases, I've seen people get injured because their egos became too heavy to lift safely. That's why, at the end of each chapter of the four essential lifts in this book, I've included a Do It Right portion to make sure you perform the lifts correctly and minimize your risks of getting injured.

Light Load and Off Weeks

I hardly hear of people who perform strength training exercises who lift lighter than their usual working weights on a regular basis. Probably, it's because of the belief that if heavy is good, heavier is better, and heaviest is best. However, the truth is that no one could strength-train optimally all year round!

If you push your body to do strength training at a balls-to-the-walls pace all year round, your body will mount a coup to force you to give it a break every now and then. The scary part is if your body does it for you, chances are it'll be in the form of getting sick or worse, getting injured. So do yourself a favor by reducing the amount of weight you lift for a week every one or two months. Even better, why not schedule a week off from strength training at least once every four to six months to give your muscles more time to recuperate and recover? Kevin Levrone, one of the greatest bodybuilders in history, took a couple of weeks off every year to let his muscles recover and optimize the results of his strength training program.

Conditioning Workouts

Many people assume that aerobic and anaerobic or resistance training programs are mutually exclusive and that they can't coexist. Nothing can be farther from the truth. Endurance athletes – people who do mostly aerobic training – benefit by incorporating even just a small amount of strength training to their regimen, knowing that stronger muscles can lead to increased endurance. Therefore, you can also maximize your strength training gains by incorporating some aerobic or conditioning workouts into your strength training regimen.

Conditioning workouts are also an important part of a good strength training program because you'll need to have enough anaerobic capacity, i.e., a large enough "gas" tank, to be able to hoist the heaviest weights possible for the optimal number of repetitions and sets. If you have very poor conditioning, you won't be able to lift heavy and long enough to build muscle and burn fat. Good examples of conditioning workouts that you can incorporate in your strength training regimen include hill sprints, running, biking, brisk walking on an inclined treadmill, skipping rope, or using the Stairmaster for at least

30 minutes twice or thrice weekly at moderate to high intensity.

20

Chapter 3 - The Essential Lifts

The best reason for getting into a strength training program is for building muscle and burning body fat. There are many different strength training routines that can help you achieve those goals, but all of them have a common thread: essential lifts or exercises. These essentials work well for most people because they target the most number of muscles and burn the most calories and body fat during execution. These essential lifts include:

1. Squats;
2. Deadlifts;
3. Overhead Presses; and
4. Bench Presses.

These exercises are called compound or multi-joint exercises, which involve several muscle groups when it comes to proper execution. The reason why compound exercises are the best for building muscle mass and burning body fat is that you recruit more muscle cells when performing them, which means the more energy used, the more calories and fat burned. For each of these exercises, a very good place to start would be 3 working sets of 12 repetitions each, with only 30 seconds of rest in between sets. The brief resting period ensures that your heart rate stays elevated for optimal fat burning and workout intensity for muscle building.

Isolation exercises are the opposite of compound or multi-joint exercises, i.e., they involve only one body part or muscle group. Isolation exercises are very good additions or supplementary exercises to a good strength training program, and they can be added or removed as the need arises. Compound exercises, like the four essential ones we'll discuss, are the meat and potatoes of a good strength training program, and the only things you can change with them are repetitions, weight, and pace.

Chapter 4 - Squats

This is considered as the alpha dog of all strength training exercises. Why? It's because the squat is the exercise that recruits the most number of muscle groups, where the biggest lower body muscles and core muscles are highlighted, and as we've discussed earlier, the more muscle groups you involve in an exercise, the more body fat and calories you can burn. Squats are an indispensable part of any serious strength training program.

One of the best features of the squat exercise is that it can be performed with very heavy weight, very light weight, or no weight at all (bodyweight only). If you perform bodyweight squats, you won't need any equipment, and you can do it anytime and anywhere!

Why You Should Perform Squats

One of the benefits of including squats – whether bodyweight or weighted – is better athletic performance, particularly for sports that require explosive running or jumping action, such as basketball, volleyball, sprints, and American football. Squats, when properly done, can help you jump higher and run faster. For this reason, squats are an indispensable part of many professional sports training programs.

Another benefit of including the king of all strength training exercises in your program is a balanced and mobile body. As you age, your ability to stay as mobile and balanced as you are now is highly dependent on the strength of your legs and core muscles. Given that squats primarily work out your leg and core muscles, performing this exercise consistently can help you stay as mobile and balanced later on in life.

And speaking of maintaining mobility and balance, squats can also help you reduce your risks for injuries due to accidental falls or sports activities. Many falls or sports-related injuries happen because of weak connective tissues, ligaments, and stabilizer muscles – all of which can be strengthened with squats. To a great extent, performing squats properly can also help you minimize injuries through improved flexibility, particularly in the leg and feet areas. The motions involved in performing squats can improve your hips, ankles, and knees' ranges of motion.

Last but not the least, squats can give you a tight butt and waistline. How? For one, it burns the most calories and, consequently, body fat. Less body fat means a tighter butt and waistline. More than just burning more fat, squats help build muscle in your legs and buns, which fill them out and make them appear toned and shapely!

Optimizing Your Squat Benefits through Variety

You can perform squats in several different ways in order to zone in on different areas of your leg muscles. For example, performing front squats focuses on working out your thigh or quadriceps muscles (quads). Back squats bring to play more muscles in your legs, including the butt and hamstring muscles, and as such, it is the better squat variation for optimizing muscle mass and fat burning.

Another way you can change things up during squats and optimize your results is to change the width of your stance. A wider stance will help work out your butt and hamstring muscles more, a sumo wrestler-like stance will work out your adductor muscles, too, and a narrow stance will focus more on your thigh or quad muscles.

Lastly, you can change things up with your squat routine by using different pieces of equipment apart from barbells, such as kettlebells, Swiss balls, dumbbells, and even just your body weight. However, if you want consistently superior results, you should do most of your squats using barbells. Speaking of barbells, you can go free weight or use a Smith machine. The free weight version is superior to the Smith machine one, but it doesn't mean you can't use the Smith machine. You can incorporate it as a supplementary squat workout, such as an extra set of squats after your free weight sets for optimally maxing out your legs or as an occasional substitute for free weights, especially when you're not in optimal condition.

Do It Right

As mentioned in the previous chapter, proper form is crucial for reaping the benefits of any of the essential – and even the non-essential – lifts. More importantly, using proper form will minimize your risks of getting injured. Here's how to squat properly:
  - Whether you're using a barbell, a dumbbell, a Smith machine, or your bodyweight, start by bringing your hips as far back as possible.

- Always remember to keep your lower back straight at all times. Feel your hamstrings stretch.
- With your hips bent, start bringing your body down – keeping your lower back arched – by bending at the knees until you reach the squatting position, i.e., your hamstrings are parallel to the floor. This is the optimal squatting position for maximum weight.
- Push back up to the starting position through your heels, stopping short of locking out your knees. Do not lock your knees to ensure constant tension on your leg muscles and to minimize risks for knee injuries later on. That's one repetition.

Chapter 5 - Deadlifts

You learned earlier that the squat is the king of strength training exercises. Now, meet the queen! Actually, you can consider the deadlift to be somewhat of an equal to the squat, so depending on your preference, you can switch titles for this and the squat. However, on a more serious note, the titles really don't matter much. What's important is that this should be one of your strength training exercise staples.

The reason why the deadlift is a major component of any good strength training program is because as a compound exercise, it works several big muscle groups, including the lower back muscles, your core muscles, your hamstrings, your butt muscles, your hips, your thighs, and your forearm muscles, too! A very unique aspect of this exercise is it helps make your lower back muscles really strong and, in the process, reduces your risks for injuries. Weak lower back muscles often result in back instability, which leads to lower back problems and injuries.

You can perform this with a barbell or a pair of dumbbells. When using a barbell, you can perform this exercise using one of two grips: with both hands pronated or overhand grips or an alternate grip where one hand employs a supinated or underhand grip while the other employs a pronated one.

Why You Should Perform Deadlifts

One of the best reasons for incorporating deadlifts into your strength training program is improved posture. Performing this exercise can help you strengthen the muscles involved in your posture and stability: your core muscles. Stronger core muscles help you maintain an erect posture for longer, which is important for minimizing risks for lower back injuries due to fatigue.

Another benefit to doing this exercise is it can make your grip stronger. This is because you need strong forearm muscles, i.e., grip strength, to lift progressively heavier weights with deadlifts. During deadlifts, the only thing that will ensure that the barbell or dumbbells stay connected to your body and off the floor is your grip. So by progressively overloading your lower back muscles during deadlifts, you also do the same to your forearm muscles and make your grip stronger over time.

Another benefit – one that many people can't believe comes from doing deadlifts – is you get some cardiovascular or aerobic workout in. If you can't believe it too, try performing 10 repetitions of a barbell or dumbbell deadlift using a relatively heavy weight. Then tell me that it doesn't involve a good amount of aerobic or cardiovascular workout.

You can also benefit from regularly performing deadlifts by being able to lift heavier "real-life" weights. This is because compared to the other three essential exercises, most real-life lifts like bringing a heavy box of office supplies or groceries from point A to point B require strong lower back and leg muscles, as well as good grip strength.

Lastly, you minimize your risks for lower back and other back-related injuries when you regularly perform deadlifts. Given that it works your lower back, core, and leg muscles, deadlifts help make these muscles that are very important for stability, balance, and safety much stronger, which may help reduce risks of getting injured.

Do It Right

To perform the deadlift correctly, keep the following things in mind:

- Assume the same stance as you would normally do right before you jump, i.e., your leg stance should be narrow.
- As you pick up the barbell or dumbbell from the ground just before performing the lifts, make sure that your lower back's straight, your hips are down, and your shoulders are positioned directly above the knees to minimize your risks of getting injured.
- Always keep your back straight – from the moment you lift the barbell or dumbbell off the ground, to straightening your body at the top of the movement, until you lower it back down.

Chapter 6 - Overhead Press

This exercise is also known as military or shoulder presses and primarily works out your front shoulder muscles or anterior deltoids. For optimal fat burning and muscle building results, the overhead press is typically done from a standing position in order to work out as many muscles as possible aside from the front deltoids, including the core muscles, the legs, and back muscles. When done from a very inclined bench, the core, leg, and back muscles aren't engaged, which means less calories and body fat are burned.

When it comes to overhead presses, barbells are preferred over dumbbells and kettlebells. This is because using the latter pieces of equipment can lead to imbalances in terms of muscle strength and size. There are also two variations of the overhead barbell press: the front and behind-the-back versions. For beginners and intermediate level lifters, the behind-the-back overhead press isn't advised because of its higher risks for injuries due to poor form, especially when lifting relatively heavier weights.

Why You Should Perform Overhead Presses

One of the key benefits of incorporating this exercise into your strength training program is a very strong core. Athlete testing has shown that standing overhead presses tend to activate the most number of muscles compared to the seated variation, and while such testing was done using dumbbells, the same conditions hold true with overhead barbell presses versus seated barbell presses.

Performing overhead presses also have a carryover benefit to another essential lift: the bench press. Why? It's because both are upper body pressing movements that involve the front delt muscles and triceps.

Lastly, performing overhead presses can help you perform better across a good number of sports, primarily because it helps train your core from an anti-extension angle. This means that during overhead presses, you'll need to resist the temptation to hyperextend your lower back because you may tip over backward or injure your lower back. Doing this helps strengthen your deep core muscles, such as the side oblique, the abdominal, and the lower back muscles, all of which are crucial for high multi-sport performance.

Do It Right

There are only a few points to keep in mind to do this exercise right:

- Always keep your lower back straight: neither hunched forward nor hyper-extended backward. Doing this will optimize your core muscles' strength and minimize your risks for lower back injuries.
- When the barbell (or dumbbell) is at shoulder level, flare your upper back muscles, i.e., your "lats." If you do this, you'll be able to handle more weight.

Chapter 7 - Bench Press

The last essential lift of any good strength training program is the bench press, which is used to strengthen and build the chest muscles. Similar to squats, bench presses can be done in several different ways in order to target your chest area's different muscles. In particular, the flat bench press will work out your chest's middle area, the incline bench press will work out your upper chest muscles, and the decline bench press will work out your lower chest or pecs.

You can choose between a barbell and a pair of dumbbells for this exercise, but for beginners, the barbell bench press is the better variation to start with. You can also use different grips for this exercise, with each targeting specific muscles in your chest. A conventional grip, i.e., a pronated one gives a different feel for your chest muscles compared to a supinated one, though the latter is an advanced technique that's not advisable for beginners and intermediate level lifters. And lastly, a narrow barbell grip will work out your triceps more than your chest and a normal or a wider grip works out your chest more than your triceps.

Why You Should Perform Bench Presses

The primary reason why you should incorporate bench presses in your strength training program is to build more power, which is one of the best ways to measure your fitness level. By definition, power is your ability to exert strength or force over a specific distance at the fastest possible speed. Bench presses can help you increase your upper-body strength, which can prove useful in many every day and recreational activities. It also doesn't hurt that a muscular chest can make you more attractive, regardless of your gender.

If you're into running, doing bench presses can help you become a more efficient and faster runner! How? To run efficiently and quickly, you need to use optimal form. This means utilizing the right upper-body movements and posture, such as looking forward, head held up, shoulders relaxed, elbows at a 90-degree angle, an open chest, and proper arm swings.

To swing your arms more efficiently from where your elbows are behind you until your arms are forward at shoulder level, your chest muscles need to get involved. The faster and stronger you're able to do this, the less effort you'll need to run and the faster you can do it. Because bench presses are aimed to strengthen your chest muscles, they can help you swing your arms more efficiently as you run, leading to faster times and less effort.

Do It Right

To perform a barbell bench press properly, here are some very important things to keep in mind:
- Begin with your head lifted slightly off from the bench.
- Grab the barbell, and use it to bring your upper body off the bench so you can position yourself correctly, i.e., the barbell should be between eye and nose level.
- Press your butt on the bench and arch your lower back.

— Bring your shoulder blades close together and your shoulders drawn back, and keep it so from the moment you lift the barbell off the rack, to when you lower it down to your chest, and until you push it back up. This will ensure that most of the stress will be on your chest muscles and not on your front shoulder muscles.

Conclusion

Thank you for buying this book. Now that you know what strength training is, its general benefits, the essential lifts of a good strength training program, and the benefits of each of the essential lifts, it's time to make a decision. Will you or will you not embark on a strength training program? It's my hope that through this book, I was able to encourage you to take action and enroll in a legit strength training program so you can build muscle, burn body fat, and get into the best shape of your life!

Thank you, and remember to share how well these strength training tips work for you. You can do that here...

Thank you,

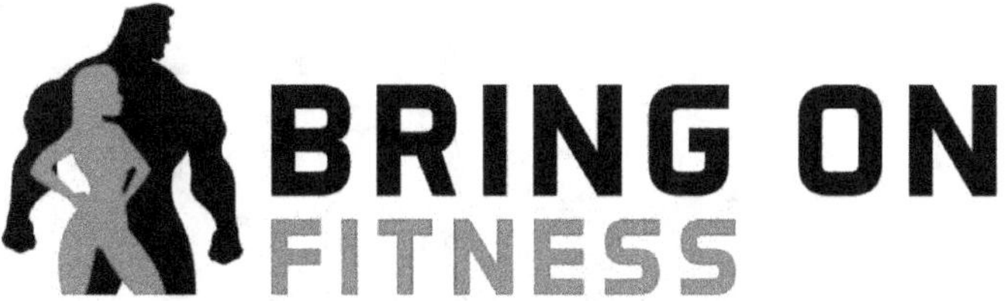

References:

https://www.everydayhealth.com/fitness/add-strength-training-to-your-workout.aspx
http://next-level-athletics.com/5-key-elements-effective-strength-program/
https://www.bodybuilding.com/content/essential-8-exercises-to-get-ripped.html
https://fitness.mercola.com/how-to-do-squats.aspx
https://www.lifehack.org/articles/lifestyle/benefits-deadlifts-you-probably-never-knew.html
https://www.livestrong.com/article/98767-benefits-bench-presses/

About Bring On Fitness

Our passion for fitness gave life to **Bring On Fitness**. We started with the goal of helping as many people as we can. To educate, motivate and to help change peoples lives for the better. Bring On Fitness is not only for the fitness enthusiasts, but also for the beginner. We strongly believe nothing is more important than learning the basics and creating a strong foundation in both nutrition - through meal planning, and in exercise - by following a specific plan. This is just as important for the beginner, as it is for the experienced athlete.

We set high standards for ourselves, the information we share, and the products we carry. Our goal is to provide you with exceptional products that suit your needs and the knowledge and motivation to help you work towards and achieve your health and fitness goals.

Keep up to date by liking us on Facebook and Instagram @bringonfitness

And for a complete list of reads and a FREE GIFT check us out at: www.bringonfitness.com

"Our Mission is to have a positive impact in changing peoples lives. We will deliver the best possible fitness and nutrition solutions that will empower people to achieve their health and fitness goals."

www.ingramcontent.com/pod-product-compliance
Lightning Source LLC
Chambersburg PA
CBHW070059260726
48658CB00002B/917